Don't Be Stupid about Stomach Acid

DontBeStupid.club Answers to Reflux, GERD, Heartburn... whatever you call it

H. Granville James

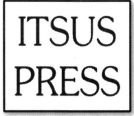

ITSUS PRESS

Don't Be Stupid about Stomach Acid
DontBeStupid.club Answers to Reflux, GERD,
Heartburn...whatever you call it

Copyright © 2016 ITSUS Press. First edition March 2016.
Illustration by the author. All rights reserved.

ISBN: 1530749883
ISBN-13: 978-1530749881

Contents

1.
Let's Begin

GERD, HEARTBURN, ACID REFLUX, whatever you call it...

Sixty million people know it hurts. You don't need us to tell you that. But we want you to know up front:

"We feel your pain".

We had it bad. That burning in your chest, coughing after eating, belching, fear of eating a big meal like on Thanksgiving, all those fun symptoms; we had reflux bad, and occasionally we still have to fight with it.

But it doesn't have to be a big deal. If you understand it, dealing with reflux is just like dealing with any of the other little injuries that become part of your life. Reflux doesn't have to torment you all the time if you're just not stupid about it. Unfortunately, we see a lot of people being stupid about it.

We've made it our mission to think about problems critically and help others do it too. We hope to eliminate the stupidity. That doesn't always make the problem disappear completely, but it is amazing how much smaller a problem can become once the stupidity is removed. Maybe all of us can be a little less stupid about reflux. Let's give it a try anyway.

We are not going to offer any secret formula or tricks. We just apply the DontBeStupid.club critical thinking principles to the discussion on GERD, Heartburn, Acid Reflux, reflux... what should we call it anyway?

Please don't bother us with the arcane medical dictionary

differences between all the terms. Yeah, we get it. They don't mean exactly the same thing. Who cares. Bottom line, it's a progression that starts at a little indigestion and ends with us dying of esophageal cancer.

Dwelling on irrelevant distinctions violates our *Don't Be Distracted* principle (see DontBeStupid.club for a detailed look at our principles and critical thinking methods. In this book the principles will be in *italics* to identify them.)

Being distracted by multiple names and definitions is one of the fundamental techniques used to keep us stupid. Fight it. Unless the distinction changes the conclusions it's irrelevant. You say "toe-may-toe", they say "toe-mah-toe". Who cares. Do you like the sauce or not?

It is far more productive (and far less stupid) if we talk about stopping the reflux progression instead of naming the many different levels.

For this book we will use reflux because it's short and easy to read. But we'll probably slip a few times and call it one of the other names too. Reflux is a good word to remember for your Scrabble game too. It's really in the dictionary and not a proper name. GERD is not acceptable on a Scrabble board.

We'll talk about food a little because it's hard to upset your stomach without it. But this is not a diet book. We're not going to offer reflux-free recipes. And we won't tell you to avoid stuff that tastes good. With apologies to all who don't eat pork, bacon is more important than reflux.

In this book, we will apply some DontBeStupid.club principles to common remedies for reflux and come up real answers. Answers you can use immediately. Answers that are free, or at least cost a lot less than what you're spending right now. Answers that are no stupid.

The best thing about answers? You don't need refills. Learn once, use forever. Answers are the cheapest medicine out there.

Will DontBeStupid.club critical thinking work for your reflux? Probably. We're going to take 10 shots at reflux here. It will be hard to miss every time. And we're pretty sure you spent less on this book than for a bottle of antacids, so there is likely a decent payback on your investment.

You will have to actually do something with the answers though. Just knowing them won't matter unless you put in a little effort. And we mean very little effort. We've done everything in this book and none of it was hard work.

We don't expect to cure the whole reflux problem here. And this is not a comprehensive medical discussion. This is a practical discussion of 10 readily available remedies for reflux using DontBeStupid.club principles as our guide.

We don't try to change the world. Just take small steps in the right direction. Following every suggestion in this book costs virtually nothing; not much time, and you'll probably save some money over whatever you're doing now. So what's to lose except some heartburn?

Here's our effort at making the world a little less stupid about acid reflux. GERD. Heartburn. Whatever...

2.
What is Acid Reflux?

DEFINE THE TARGET is a fundamental DontBeStupid.club principle. So we need to start with a quick review.

Everyone has seen something like this before. You've probably seen it look more complicated because someone thinks that makes them look smart. In keeping with the DontBeStupid.club principle of *Simplify*, this is the clearest description of what happens when you suffer with acid reflux:

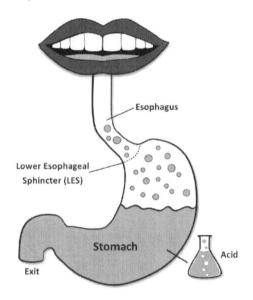

That's all it is. Acid from your stomach moving up to places it's not supposed to go. Those places are not meant to handle acid. It causes damage so your body sends you a pain signal. The body is not stupid.

Please know, your heart is not burning. The top of your stomach/lower part of your throat are in the same vicinity as your heart, so the pain comes from the same area; the confusion is obvious. They even get it confused in emergency rooms. Emergency rooms can get very stupid. But your heart is not on fire. It's not even interested, really.

Now this next part is where an awful lot of people get stupid. Even starting with a perfectly clear understanding of what is reflux, people veer off the critical thinking path and get stupid here. This is important:

Your stomach is supposed to produce acid. A lot of it. Enough acid to quickly turn that steak dinner you just ate into mush where all the nutrients can be sucked out very easily. You need the acid in your stomach, or the food cannot keep your body alive. *Respect Nature.* The stomach's natural state is low pH.

Quick review. *There Will Be Math.* pH is a measure of acidity or alkalinity relative to a neutral midpoint. The scale runs from 1 to 14. Under 7 is acid, over 7 is alkaline.

Now *There Will Be Math* even a little more than usual to make a point here. Don't run away, we'll try to make this fun. (Math kills stupidity, always fun, but that's another book.)

The pH scale is a logarithmic scale, not a linear one. Each number reflects a difference of 10 times the next number. A pH of 5 is ten times more acidic than a pH of 6. Each step is an order of magnitude bigger than the one next to it.

Logarithmic scales are used to collapse large differences into a more easily managed size. You could show the same pH information on a linear scale, but you'd have to write out the number associated with 14 to the 10th power... a little more than 289 billion. So instead of 289 billion lines, we use a pH scale that has 14.

A log scale is much easier, right? But it does diminish the perceived magnitude of the difference from one line to the next, unless you remember it's a log scale. Not linear. For the pH scale, remember the distance from one end to the other is 289 billion, not 14.

We hope that diversion into logs was a little fun. And if you found yourself enjoying it, visit our website for a lot more math. We find all of it pretty entertaining.

OK, back to stomach pH.

A healthy stomach pH is generally between 1.5 and 3. A neutral number would be 7. Remember it's a logarithmic scale? A healthy stomach pH is over 9 million times more acidic than a neutral stomach.

9 Million is a big number. If neutral is one inch, then a healthy stomach is over 140 miles away.

That was a lot of numbers for a chapter talking about reflux. We have a tendency to do that... so we'll just stop here and get back to the important point we wanted to make. A healthy stomach is VERY acidic. Your stomach wants the acid. It loves it.

Acid is not the problem.

Reflux is a problem only when acid moves up out of

your stomach into your throat. Let's always keep that distinction in mind, because a lot of being stupid starts with confusing the acid and the problem.

Gasoline in your car's tank is not a problem. The tank is built for it. But if gasoline leaves the tank via the same path it goes in, that's a big problem.

Reflux is about acid in the esophagus. In your throat. Stomach acid is not supposed to be there. And that's the condition we're fighting against.

The DontBeStupid.club Summary:

- You need a lot of acid in your stomach to digest your food.

- A healthy stomach is 9 million times more acidic than a neutral one.

- Reflux is about acid moving up out of the stomach.

- (Log scales are fun.)

3.
Answer 1: Purple Pills, Antacids, Acid Blockers, More Purple Pills

WE HAVE TO DISCUSS these products first because they're the answer most people turn to. And people spend a lot of money on them. It's a multi-billion-dollar blockbuster drug category.

Almost everyone with reflux problems tries the pill popping solution at some point. Apply the DontBeStupid.club principle *Define the Target*. Pill - a mass of medicine designed to be swallowed whole. For the purpose of this chapter's discussion, we will expand the concept to include the liquid equivalents too. They all try to do the same thing.

All of these products work toward the same goal. Whether prescription or over the counter, it doesn't matter what arcane principle it works on, they all try to do the same thing. Some block acid production, some are alkaline compounds trying to cancel out the acid already in there. Whatever their method... the result they pursue is a less acidic stomach.

Now if you read the last chapter, your DontBeStupid.club *Common Sense* bell has to be ringing in your head a little already. Being highly acid is your stomach's natural state of existence. Without that acid, you cannot digest your food. So why are we taking pills to stop that?

The most obvious principle that violates is *Respect Nature*. But to answer the question "Why?" we're going to jump right into our *Follow the Money* principle.

Reflux hurts physically, we all know that. But when dealing with physical pain, we may not spend much time thinking about how it hurts our wallet too.

Medicare pays out over $2.5 billion annually for Nexium alone, plus another $600 million for similar generics. Add another $20 billion or so for all the over the counter treatments, Tums, Rolaids, Alka-Seltzer, and on and on, and before you know it we're talking about some serious cash. Treatment for Reflux is a big business.

There is no reliable single number, and we've seen some truly stupid sounding estimates over $100 billion. *There Will Be Math*. But it's roughly a $25 billion market in the USA alone. The USA accounts for maybe 5% of the world's population. So upon analysis, maybe $100 billion isn't so stupid after all. In fact, $100 billion is too low. (Math really is fun.)

No matter what your choice among the estimates, the financial incentives for people selling treatments are clearly huge. And you pay for it, again and again. Every refill. Every trip to the drugstore. Every roll of cherry flavored antacid. This is a major cash cow for product sellers.

Did you know there are competing brands specifically marketed to children now too? Bubblegum flavored with happy cartoon kids all over the box. That's just stupid. And if you want to double the stupidity, there are prescription strength versions for kids too. Still bubblegum or cherry flavored, of course.

Even if you and your kids don't take the expensive prescriptions, someone you know probably does. And their insurance pays for it.

Even if you don't suffer with reflux at all... maybe you're reading this to help someone else... that does not save you. You are paying too. Your insurance covers it whether you use it or not. Insurance covers everyone, that's how insurance works.

And then people spend another $5 or $10 a week on over the counter remedies too.

With so much money at stake, and that money coming in on such a reliable schedule, we would be stupid to think anyone offering remedies has much interest in beating this problem. They have a good thing going.

You do something every day that causes pain, and you buy their product for relief. You do it over and over into infinity. This is a beautiful business plan. Who would mess with that?

Follow the Money. Pill providers would rather see you having chili dogs for breakfast, all you can eat, every day. They don't want you doing or learning anything that might hurt their profit. They want the cash, and don't even mind using your kids to get it.

Why do we spend so much money for such poor results? Probably more than one reason. But the biggest one is stupidity.

The DontBeStupid.club principle of *Respect Nature* should guide us here. It shouldn't even be necessary to follow the money to know pills of various colors are stupid. (Quick review of the principle: Most of the time, nature knows best. We need it more than it needs us. Visit DontBeStupid.club for more.)

So is it smart or stupid to stop the stomach from doing what nature intended?

Sometimes it's necessary to interrupt your body's natural process. If you cut yourself deeply enough, it's important to interrupt the natural process of bleeding to death. So it would be stupid to suggest you should never interrupt your body.

But *Trust Common Sense*. Just as you'd never use a tourniquet for a paper cut, you don't want to use any remedy that causes more damage than the condition being treated. Take a look at the side effects warnings. It doesn't matter what pill you look at, they all have side effects and warnings. A quick read of those warnings gives common sense a chance to kick in with an opinion. You have to *Think for Yourself*, but the drug companies are helping you out a little. Labeling laws make them do it.

OK, but sometimes you've just got to have relief. The fact is, interrupting your digestive process once in a while is not going to hurt you. Odds are very good the chili dog was not health food anyway, so you're not exactly missing out on a nutritional bonanza by not digesting it properly.

Down the line, of course, the rest of your digestive systems will have to deal with things that should have been taken care of in the stomach. Those symptoms can also be unpleasant. *Respect Nature*. Don't be surprised if altering the stomach's action causes other problems later on. You're interrupting a process that includes many steps. One thing leads to another...

Even if you only interrupt your digestion process once in a while, it's worth remembering that it's all one big chain reaction. It starts when you put something in your mouth, and it isn't over until it exits the other end. If the stomach is interrupted, something else has to take on the burden. Trading a pain in your throat for a pain somewhere else is not really progress. And it shouldn't come as a surprise unless you're stupid.

If you occasionally get the relief you need by taking a pill, great. The body is adaptable and well equipped to deal with the occasional interruption of its routines. Most likely no harm done as long as the interruption is rare. But always we must *Respect Nature*. The more you fight with nature, the more likely you are going to lose sooner or later.

Think about the difference between a good night's sleep, and a night where something wakes you up every hour. You just feel bad in the morning. Digestion is also a process that benefits from not being interrupted. Interrupt any of your body's natural processes too often, and you will feel bad.

By the way, if you do read the prescription warnings, you will find even the drug companies tell you their pills are for short term use. Their pills are not to become part of your regular diet. They say that because they have to. Nobody but you can actually enforce it. Drug companies will sell you, and your kids, as much as you will buy. Don't Be Stupid.

One last word. If you are on a prescription and decide to stop taking meds, don't be stupid and quit all at once. Your body is accustomed to being drugged right now. Just like heroin, you need to wean yourself slowly.

At this point, lawyers are much happier if we say talk to your doctor before making any changes to your meds. So do that. But don't let them talk you out of it.

The DontBeStupid.club Summary:

- Pills are very big business. A whole lot of people want you to keep buying.

- Use pills as a last resort. Make sure it's worth it. They interrupt the body's natural process. And it would be stupid to do that too often.

4.
Answer 2: Go for a Walk

YOUR REFLUX IS telling you there is more going on in your stomach than it can handle. Your stomach is literally overflowing. Pushing back. Reflux! Your body is screaming at you for help.

Don't have a stomach pump handy? (one big reflux.) No Roman Vomitorium nearby? (Those are a myth anyway. They were never nearby...)

You want to clear out your stomach fast? Go for a walk.

Just go for a walk after any challenging meal. Or anytime your reflux is acting up. Get up and walk.

Does this work?

Let's *Define the Target* a little. Walk – Move at a regular pace by lifting and setting down each foot in turn. In bipeds, never having both feet off the ground at once. So we're talking about a nice walk here, not about sprints or running a marathon. In fact, a marathon likely would aggravate your reflux. (Side note to marathoners suffering with reflux: try half marathons for a while and see if you notice improvement.)

Your body is a big pump. When you move, it pumps. Everything inside tends to move around getting to where it's supposed to go. This happens whenever you move naturally.

The body does not have an on-off switch. Movement provides the stimulus, the push for everything to work. Within normal life activity boundaries, the more you move the more efficiently your body works. And if you don't move, the body never turns on. And pretty soon you die.

If you can take a nice 20-minute walk after a challenging meal, in most cases you get relief. Just walk around the block, or walk around the house, or if you have a treadmill serving as a clothes hanger.... if you can just manage to do a little walking, then you are very likely to experience results faster than any tablet can deliver in that same amount of time.

The added bonus? You're helping nature and not fighting with it. Your body wants to pump. Your stomach wants to make acid to consume the overload of food you just sent it. Your body wants to empty the stomach, and it wants to pump the nutrients to the proper destinations.

Give it a little help. *Respect Nature*. Don't kill the acid. Walk instead. This is a habit for us now. As soon as we realize we ate a little too much, or too rich, we just head out for a walk. Never a problem.

The rest of your digestive system appreciates the walk too. One very effective way to help everything exit in the right direction is to make sure the path is available. That path has to be available so the contents of your stomach can exit when ready. Keep the pump going. If the path is not open, the alternate path of least resistance just might be up the throat instead. Yuck.

The side effects from walking are considerably

different from the side effects of pills. If you were going to advertise prescription walking, the list of possible side effects would make you smile, not scare you. (Even though your heart was never burning it appreciates walking too. But that's another book.)

The DontBeStupid.club Summary:

- Walking helps, respects nature, and it doesn't cost any money.

- Get up and pump.

5.
Answer 3: Slippery Elm Bark

SLIPPERY ELM BARK is a not-so-secret ingredient that is as close as you will come to a miracle cure. We know this one works because it's a personal favorite. You mix it with some liquid, plain hot water works if you're boring, and you drink it.

We know it's not-so-secret because you can buy it on Amazon Prime. Even organic, it can be at your door in two days. Or maybe within the hour the way Amazon is going. Alexa might even know when you're thinking about it.

Apply the DontBeStupid.club principle *Define the Target*. Bark – The tough protective outer sheath of a trunk or branch.

Slippery elm bark is exactly what it sounds like, the bark of an elm tree. And the product we eat is the inner layer of the bark. The Slippery Elm varietal has the thickest layer and, therefore, yields the most product, but basically the inner layer of bark from any elm tree has the same properties.

We can do a whole book on just Elm Bark, but that's not the point here. Just buy it from a reputable producer, organic whenever possible, and you don't have to worry about it.

But if you're looking for entertaining reading, we really enjoy the stories of how George Washington's troops lived on Slippery Elm bark. That's right, Slippery Elm bark is one big reason why the USA is not still part of the British Empire.

All we want today is for you to consider elm bark might help with your reflux. Nothing so grand as the birth of a nation. But if it was good enough for George and his troops... we're just sayin', maybe you can think about it too.

Let's move into the evaluation. We said Slippery Elm can be a miracle cure. And it really can. We've given away many bags to suffering friends and they think we're heroes. We've seen it over and over. But people can get very stupid about it. We've seen that over and over too.

Respect Nature. You can buy the pure product, powdered and bagged. Just the bark, powdered and bagged. It's pretty cheap too, especially compared to purple pill prescriptions.

You can buy the simple product, or you can choose from dozens of different variations. More expensive of course. And usually of diminished quality. Let's *Follow the Money*.

For a benchmark, let's use our favorite organic brand of powdered bark. It's about $29 for a one-pound bag. *There Will Be Math*. That's one pound, 16 ounces, 453.59 grams or 453,592 milligrams. About $1.81 per ounce. Don't worry about where to buy it right now, there's a link at the very end of the book. But we don't want to distract you from critical thinking right now.

Slippery Elm Powder, pure, organic. $1.81 per ounce.

Potions and extracts made from Slippery Elm cost $5 to upwards of $10 per ounce. What's in them? Depends on which supplier, but they always contain one or more of the following: water, vegetable oil, sugar syrup, and occasionally a little alcohol (that makes it feel like medicine when you put it on your tongue, *Don't Be Distracted*).

Frequently some "glycerin" is in there too. It sounds medicinal. Glycerin is really just something left after oils break down. Basically, it's the garbage that's left after many different processes involving fats. But thanks to modern science, now commercial uses abound. It's used in antifreeze and hand lotion among other things, and pills too of course.

Side note for you vegetarians, glycerin is often derived from animal fat. Not sure what's ok in your hand lotion, but you probably don't want to eat it. Most everybody, even carnivores, react poorly to ingesting large quantities of glycerin. So we'd actually recommend no one eat it.

All of the additional ingredients in these "elixirs" are very cheap, they have no health benefit, but they help make slippery elm bark taste and feel more expensive in your mouth. These added ingredients also bulk up the size of the container. So it looks like it's worth more, but you get less of the product you really want, the slippery elm bark. Spend more, get less. That's stupid.

A best-selling potion, not the most expensive, is $26 for 4 ounces. Roughly four times the cost of powder, and not even 4 pure ounces of the product you want. The slippery elm is cut with other ingredients that do nothing for your stomach; the best you can hope for is that they are inert. But you paid extra for them in any case.

Tablets are generally cheaper than potions and usually consist mostly of the bark. Basically, the powder is compressed under high pressure into a tablet. 100 tablets of 400 milligrams each costs around $5. It makes a nice sized bottle with plenty of room for very serious looking labels. (You can pay a lot more, we've seen bottles over $30, but we're trying to be fair here.)

This best-selling tablet example we'll use is $5 for a bottle totaling 40,000 milligrams. *There Will Be Math.* We have more than ten times that amount, 453,592 milligrams in our $29 bag of powder. So this tablet option works out to be almost twice the price. But at least we're not paying for any glycerin.

Even if you want to pay almost twice as much to have your powder made into tablet, the compression process causes heat high enough to alter the nature of the product. And if nothing else, it will take longer to dissolve in your stomach. Seems stupid to pay extra for making it less effective.

As you look through all the various ways you might buy Slippery Elm Bark, if you find one where the alterations and extra expense adds any value, please let us know. In our experience, variations exist primarily for the purpose of extracting more money from the buyer, and they give you less of the actual product for your money. Don't Be Stupid.

In all cases, these tablet and potion variations miss out

on one of the main benefits to slippery elm. One of the ways Slippery Elm works is as a simple physical barrier. Once mixed with liquid, it forms a viscous layer on top of whatever it lands on. Plop some on the counter and you'll see what we mean. When you drink it, it coats the surface of your throat protecting it from acid and other abuses. And it lands on top of whatever went into your stomach before.

(Have you ever put aloe gel over a burn? Same thing. Actually, Slippery Elm poultice is used as an effective treatment for burns too.)

The best way to take the powder is mixed with liquid, forming a thick drink. If you're hard-core you can just stir it into a glass of warm water and chug it.

This method preserves one of the most important benefits. When mixed with liquid into a "tea", the slippery elm layer on top of what's already in your stomach tends to keep things in place. It is very difficult for stomach acid to move up through the slippery elm barrier and get into your throat. The barrier keeps it in the stomach, where it belongs. Pills and potions can't do that.

In many cases, relief with Slippery Elm bark tea is almost instant, much faster than an antacid tablet can dissolve. And with no unnatural side effects. Slippery elm is just real food. You can live on it. Try this:

Slippery Elm "Tea" Recipe

Ingredients:

- cup full of very hot water
- 2T organic Slippery Elm powder. Use less if you

must. Even a little will do some good.

- Small amount of natural sweetener. Stevia for zero calories but maple syrup or honey work great too.

- ½ tsp vanilla extract (optional. Yeah, we know it's an extract. But it's 1/2 teaspoon and real vanilla beans are expensive.)

- Big shake of cinnamon (also optional, but yummy)

Directions: throw everything into a blender and whiz it up. Put it back in that cup and drink it.

Is it tea? Not really. Ok, it's more like a slimy porridge. But if it works for you, it will start looking more and more beautiful every day.

And seriously, if you pig out on something you know causes heartburn, just finish with a slippery elm tea chaser. Remember, you want it on top of all that acid in your stomach.

The DontBeStupid.club Summary:

- Try Slippery Elm Bark.

- Use the whole powder from a bag and mix your own drink.

- It's cheap, does not interfere with your body's normal functions, and has health benefits even beyond keeping your stomach acid in place.

- It can keep you alive through a Valley Forge winter.

6.
Answer 4: Don't Use the Dishwasher

THIS IS REALLY about gravity. But you can't load the dishwasher without gravity being involved, and everyone needs a good excuse to postpone doing the dishes.

Define the Target. Gravity - the force of nature that causes anything with mass to move toward the center of the Earth. Defying gravity violates the *Respect Nature* principle.

Yes, we know airplanes and rocket ships defy gravity. But if you have any doubt that's fighting with nature, just look at the energy required to get a few feet off the ground.

Reflux is about the acid getting up out of your stomach and into your throat. In our normal relationship with the center of the Earth, gravity is helping keep the acid in your stomach. And any form of bending over changes gravity into one of the factors working against us.

Now please don't get too involved with all the nonsense you've heard about one-way valves at the top of your stomach, valves that break, or any other such nonsense that supposedly makes you immune to gravity if your body is just working right.

You are not broken if you respond to gravity. And you

should not rush to spend money with those who would be so happy to fix you for a fee.

You have a sphincter at the top of your stomach/bottom of your throat. This is not a one-way valve, it's a sphincter. It's remarkably similar to the sphincter at your other end, the final exit, that you get familiar with on a daily basis. Well... a daily basis if your stomach has enough acid and is doing its job.

Imagine using that lower "exit" sphincter while standing on your head. Gravity would have some effect, right? It works that way at the top of your stomach too. Everything that weighs anything is going to flow toward the center of the Earth.

Gravity doesn't care about acid reflux. If your throat gets between the center of the earth and your stomach, then your stomach acid is going to flow through your throat. Gravity can be friend or foe. And nature doesn't care which you choose. Rivers only flow downhill.

Depending on many factors, some people's sphincters are stronger than others. In cases of extreme weakness, there are surgeries that sometimes make a sphincter hold back a little more. But we mean extreme weakness here with a capital E. There is wide variation in "normal" sphincter leakage and surgery is not a correction for the normal effects of gravity.

There are also hiatal hernias. This is simply a condition where part of the stomach is sticking up through the sphincter into your esophagus. These are remarkably common, and obviously can make acid reflux a bigger problem.

And, of course, there are expensive surgical fixes for

hiatal hernias too. But you would be stupid to not try everything else first. Anything that requires anesthesia is a last resort. And we want to stick with answers you can use immediately here. This chapter is about gravity, not surgery.

Gravity isn't always the bad guy. You can use gravity to help a hiatal hernia sometimes. As we said, in a hiatal hernia the top part of the stomach has been pushed up where it is not meant to be. You might be able to use gravity to move your stomach back down. And that will help with reflux. See "Bonus Content" below.

So don't load the dishwasher after eating. If you bend over, the sphincter at the top of your stomach now has gravity to add on to the list of all the other challenges in trying to keep stomach contents where they belong. With proper caution, that sphincter can even adjust for a hiatal hernia. But it is not accustomed to adding the force of gravity into the list of its challenges.

Stand on your head with a full stomach, and it's going to leak into your throat. It's not your sphincter's fault, or a weak valve of some kind. It's just gravity. And ignoring it is just stupid.

Of course we understand most people are not stupid enough to eat a huge burrito then go stand on their head. But do they load the dishwasher? If you have any acid reflux symptoms, you're better off having another beer instead.

See? Gravity can be a force for good. It can be a great excuse for drinking beer instead of doing the dishes.

The DontBeStupid.club Summary:

- Using gravity to your advantage usually helps.

- Gravity provides a great reason to avoid chores and have a beer.

- It's free. It's a force of nature.

Bonus Content - The Hiatal Hernia exercise:

Helps some people. At worst it's harmless and you might entertain anyone watching.

First thing in the morning, drink a glass of warm water. Stretch your arms out wide, rise up on your toes and thump down hard on your heels 5 times. Then reach your arms over your head and pant fast 10 times. That's it. The warm water will give your stomach some weight, the thumping on your heels encourages your stomach to drop down, and the panting exercises your diaphragm to tighten it back up. If you have osteoporosis or disc problems in your back Don't Be Stupid, skip this exercise; thumping down on your heels is a bad idea if your bones can't take it.

7.
Answer 5: Smoking

THIS ONE IS your comedic interlude.

If you're a smoker, and the risks of various cancers and heart disease, etc., have not made you quit, then it's stupid for us to suggest a little heartburn will cause you to kick the habit. So have a laugh on us.

But if you need one more reason, just in case this is the straw that breaks the camel's back, here it is:

Smokers are way more likely to have acid reflux symptoms than non-smokers. Pick your study, we don't need to worry over whether it's three times or ten times more likely, or which study is more scientifically verifiable. *Simplify*. Smoking is strongly linked to acid reflux. Quitting will help.

Chewing tobacco is worse by the way. It delivers more nicotine to the throat and stomach. It might be better for your lungs, but it's worse for your acid reflux.

If you are among the roughly half of smokers who are stressed out over their smoking, then you're doing double damage. Stress is bad for your reflux. So you get a double shot of bad that way, stress and the actual smoking. If you're going to smoke, at least relax and enjoy it.

And now for the trifecta. Smokers spend a lot of money

on smoking. If you are ever short of funds, stressed about it and smoking, you are a just a reflux machine. You can fix a lot of problems all at once just by quitting.

It's easy to postpone quitting. Especially if the money doesn't bother you. Most of the other problems take years to show up. There is no immediate reward for quitting today. But reflux hurts RIGHT NOW. You can start feeling better right now. Why wait?

If you are a smoker with reflux, you're actually lucky. Smokers without reflux don't have the immediate incentive you do. Anyone who quits today might live longer, but that comes later. You can relieve some pain immediately, right now today. That's real motivation.

So we hate to be yet another of those annoying people who tells you to quit smoking. But you have to admit, the argument isn't stupid. We're not suggesting you quit so you can live to be 100. We're just saying live better right now.

The DontBeStupid.club Summary:

- Quitting smoking helps and saves money too.

- But you already knew that.

8.
Answer 6: Medications and Supplements

HOW IRONIC. The treatment you're using for something else also causes or contributes to your reflux.

You can't read all the warnings and disclaimers about side effects from drug companies these days. The labels are too long and the print is too small. In magazine advertisements, the warnings go on for pages now. Too many warnings mean we just ignore them all. They're breaking our *Simplify* principle and they get ignored as the result.

(Don't blame the drug companies for that problem. They don't really want to write all those pages telling you what's wrong with their products. That would be stupid. They want you to buy.)

A lot of the most common drugs and supplements taken today cause, or at least contribute to, acid reflux. We are not going to do detailed pharmacology analysis here. Let's just get to an answer we can use ASAP. Apply the DontBeStupid.club principle of *Simplify*.

We see an easy division into three groups: those KNOWN to cause problems, those that MAY cause problems, and those that do not directly cause problems but contribute to the problem in other ways.

The "known to cause problems" group includes bone strengthening or osteoporosis drugs; blood pressure meds, calcium channel and beta-blockers; and Ibuprofen.

That is not all of them, but that group covers a high percentage of the drugs being taken by a whole lot of people with reflux problems. If you are on a prescription from this group, or just pop ibuprofen regularly for your aches and pains, you're probably feeding your reflux problem as well. If you take more than one, your chances go up exponentially.

There is a lot of data out there. Some studies show a little effect; some show a lot. Some drugs have been studied more than others. Some drugs have different levels of impact. *Simplify.* All of the data says something bad, it's just a question of how bad. If you take these drugs and have reflux, it's something to consider for improvement.

Follow the Money. All of the studies are funded by people who want to sell their drugs, so none are motivated to tell you the darker side of the probability. And yet they still must acknowledge there is some likelihood of reflux as a side-effect. The makes us think the true likelihood is higher than stated.

Don't Be Distracted by arguing about the statistics (see our website for a deeper statistics discussion.) Our point is simply that these drugs are known reflux triggers and dealing with that fact might help your acid reflux.

Talk to your doctor, but don't just accept an added prescription for reducing stomach acid (see Answer

#1). Make your doctor explore alternatives with you. For example, many different drugs are available to treat high blood pressure. Many choices are available. One of them may not feed your reflux problem.

In other cases, maybe they will tell you to just go for a walk (see Answer #2 and hang on to that doctor).

In all cases, the right answer is not going to be adding another prescription. *Simplify*. You want fewer pills, not more. Fewer means less chances to cause a problem.

Our "may cause problems group" includes aspirin, fish oil supplements and any sedative. Again, this is not everything, but a whole lot of people with reflux problems are impacted by this list. There are fewer studies and more *Trust Common Sense* required with this group.

Aspirin increases stomach acid without giving it something to digest. It dissipates quickly, but some people are more sensitive to it than others and may get some heartburn. If you take a lot of aspirin, especially if you take it at bedtime, try taking less and see if you notice a reduction in reflux symptoms.

Fish Oil supplements, or any concentrated fat extract, basically fool the stomach into thinking the whole piece of food is in there needing acid to digest. So you digest the supplement OK but are left with acid looking for the rest of the fish. The best answer here is to take it with a piece of bread.

Unless you have Celiac disease... but that's another book. Take your fish oil with oatmeal if you want to safely cover all the gluten bases.

Or the best bet? *Respect Nature*. Just eat the damn salmon.

Sedatives relax you and that's great. They also relax your sphincters. That's not always great. And then you lay down. And maybe you even roll over on your stomach. Get the idea? Everything is very relaxed and nothing is working to keep stomach acid where it belongs.

Sedatives don't cause reflux. But if you use them, consider how your behavior after taking them might add to the problem. Use the *Respect Nature* principle. Gravity needs to help your now very relaxed throat sphincter. And the muscles in your throat that normally push the food down are happily relaxing too. Don't let gravity push back against all those relaxing muscles. They're currently very lazy muscles and will just let the acid pass on by.

Our third group includes all the pills that people say cause them heartburn, but probably do not.

An awful lot of medications are just aggressive going down. They just irritate the soft tissue in your throat on the way down. And if you already suffer from reflux, then your throat is already more sensitive to start with.

If possible, drink a lot of water when you take something unnatural. Even better, take a shot of slippery elm tea first (see Answer #3). And stand up as straight as possible (see Answer #4). Use gravity to your advantage.

This is just *Trust Common Sense*, but becomes extra necessary because most prescription drugs are not substances your throat is naturally developed to be in contact with. Drug companies don't think much about your reflux when they make their drugs for other problems.

Just make sure whatever med you are taking does not stay in contact with your throat for too long. It's an unnatural coupling. *Respect Nature*. Your throat has never encountered most compounds made in a laboratory.

The DontBeStupid.club Summary:

- Some medications and supplements are known to cause problems.

- Some medications probably cause problems.

- Change your prescriptions or find alternate treatments if possible.

- At least make sure all of them contact your throat as little as possible. This costs nothing.

9.
Answer 6A: Pills that Work

THERE ARE SOME pill solutions available that *Respect Nature*. In virtually all cases the evidence is anecdotal, but there is *Common Sense* supporting it. Many people experience relief from these so we want to do a quick run through here.

As we age, our stomach produces less acid. It's why you could eat anything you wanted as a kid. Remember your "cast iron" stomach when you were 12? We could digest anything...It's kind of scary kids use reflux treatments today. What the hell must they be eating?

Later on, things change. By the time you're 60, your stomach is making roughly half the acid it did when you were 12. For some people, it's even less. That will make a difference in how you digest. Not many 60-year-olds still claim a "cast iron" stomach.

Adding a digestive enzyme can help.

Or maybe just eat more pineapple. The bromelain in pineapple is such a strong digestive aid that it's actually associated with diarrhea. (Better stick with just a couple pieces until you know your tolerance.)

Papain found in papayas is used as a meat tenderizer. Getting a little more papaya along with your steak can help compensate for low stomach acid.

Bromelain and papain are available as pills too. Although these extracts are not our first choice, they are readily available and not terribly expensive. They *Respect Nature*, at least a little, because they're just adding a little more help to what should be going on in your stomach anyway.

You can't really eat pineapple or papaya with every meal. So to get those benefits a concession has to be made somewhere. A few pills might be better than nothing. Just be sure to choose a product that is as pure as possible.

"Deglycyrrhizinated" licorice or DGL is a supplement that produces mucus growth in the stomach and reduces spasms. It also has a harmonizing effect on other herbs when taken together. We have more on this one later (see Answer #8).

A more direct approach is to just take a hydrochloric acid supplement. These scare us a little. They are chemically derived in a laboratory and there is not much hard data available from studying them. There is some logic to suggesting they help digestion in a stomach not producing enough acid, but we just don't have enough evidence to get comfortable.

A good probiotic also helps things along. You have a lot of beneficial bacteria in your digestive system, but exterior forces like antibiotics kill them. Fermented foods and probiotic supplements help keep this important part of your digestion in balance and doing its job.

Probiotics are primarily to benefit your intestines and are not specifically for your stomach, but it's about emptying the stomach, making room for the next load you send down. Everything has to make its way down the path to the exit and that path needs to remain open. (Wouldn't that make for a fun book?)

The DontBeStupid.club Summary:

- There are some pills that might help, like a digestive enzyme, DGL or probiotics.

- Pineapple and Papaya taste good and probably help digestion too.

- We don't like the hydrochloric acid approach.

10.
Answer 7: Overeating

How much you eat is more important than what you eat.

Here we apply the DontBeStupid.club *First Things First* principle. There is absolutely no point in worrying about what foods trigger your heartburn if you're going to eat too much. A huge bowl of healthy food is going to give you more trouble than half a chili dog.

There is more reflux on Thanksgiving than on any other day of the year. Do turkey and mashed potatoes cause heartburn? Of course not. But when you eat three days' worth with some pie for dessert, all at one sitting? Then that turkey feast is worse than a chili dog.

Overeating is the single biggest cause of heartburn. Quantity equals trouble. This is not the most popular concept to promote. And now we apply the *Follow the Money* principle again.

No one makes money if you eat less. Not the people selling the food, not the people selling the drugs, not the people selling the diet books, not the gym where you hope to lose weight. Absolutely no one profits because you eat less. No one except you.

Everywhere you turn, you are encouraged to eat more. And then treat the symptoms of reflux when you get them. Treat the symptoms but ignore the cause of the problem.

Let's apply the principle *There Will Be Math* here. The complete formula is actually quantity plus time. Your stomach is very efficient at emptying itself out. But normally it's not trying to do that instantly.

Your stomach is very good at emptying itself instantly too. But that's called puking and it's not a preferred remedy for reflux. If that happens, you really know you've gone too far.

In many cases, people eat so fast their throat and/or stomach cannot handle the quantity. Chewing more, eating slowly, and just adding more time between courses, all help reduce acid reflux.

Ever overflow a funnel by pouring into it too fast? Well, your mouth is bigger at the top than your throat is at the bottom. You can put it in the top a lot faster than it can exit at the bottom.

If it ever seems like food is sticking in your throat, it's probably not really "sticking". It's just backing up. Consider whether or not you put it in so fast it cannot pass through the sphincter and into your stomach all at once.

Or maybe you swallowed something without chewing it enough, and now it's trying to squeeze through a smaller opening to get into your stomach. It won't. It will sit at the top until it softens enough to slide through. What will soften it? Well, acid for one thing. And whatever you swallow next will be piling on top too. That throat is getting crowded, and digestion is not supposed to happen in there!

Chew longer and your saliva can do its job. *Respect Nature*. By the time the food hits your throat, the softening process should be well underway. This takes practice. When you think you're done chewing, just hang on and give it a couple more chomps. If it tastes good, like bacon, you get to enjoy it longer this way too. You are rewarded for your patience. Take your time and enjoy the food.

And, of course, it's possible to just overload your stomach. Even if you fill it slowly enough, you can still swallow faster than your stomach can empty. Digestion begins immediately, but it takes anywhere from 4 to 8 hours to get mostly finished.

Stomachs stretch, but most people feel "full" at somewhere between 1 and 1.5 liters. Stretch means it wants to shrink back again, so the more you stretch it the more it pushes back. Your digestive system including your stomach has design limits, just like every other system out there. Your car can't pull too much weight, a 750 ml bottle cannot hold a liter, and a camel's back can only hold a certain number of straws before it breaks.

When you think about eating, don't push your equipment beyond what it's designed to do. Pushing any system beyond what you know it can do is just stupid. You know it's going to break sooner or later. *Respect Nature*.

Another bonus to slower eating, you lose weight. This is inevitable. Your brain is about 15 minutes behind your stomach in knowing when it's had enough. You will eat less because you will want less, just by going slower.

Best answer, eat with someone you like talking to. Let the conversation flow. You will eat slower, and less.

The DontBeStupid.club Summary:

- Eat less and it will help.

- Eat slower and it will help.

- And you save money too.

11.
Answer 8: Licorice (or do you say Liquorice?)

WE'RE INCLUDING THIS one because it's a popular choice to treat heartburn among those into "alternative" medicines.

We're neither into or out of "alternative medicine". We're not even sure the term means anything. Medicine is a general term and the alternative would be no medicine. A lot of good doctors will tell you to eat more vegetables. That's good medicine, we're not sure if it's alternative or not.

Someday we may have to do a whole book on "alternative" medicine. It's loaded with stupidity. But for now, we just want to apply our DontBeStupid.club principles to this licorice answer for reflux.

This answer has potential for reflux but also has a lot of stupidity attached to it as well. Here we must *Define the Target* in order to avoid being stupid. Licorice/Liquorice - a legume, like beans and peas. But we don't eat the licorice fruit. We use the root.

Throughout recorded history, licorice has been chewed to help with many health conditions. More precisely, licorice plant root has been chewed. King Tut's tomb was loaded with the stuff. Maybe Tut had acid reflux...

Licorice is abundant, cheap, and mostly used to make cigarettes. That's a little ironic since we've already identified smoking as a cause of acid reflux (see Answer #5). But licorice extract makes cigarettes smell and taste better, and delivers a more pleasant smoking experience. It keeps things moist and it does other nice things too like relax airway passages. But let's not digress too far into why licorice is great for smoking.

Licorice extract is also in some over the counter cough medicines. The relaxing passages thing? Helps you stop coughing too.

You know where there is no licorice? In "Licorice". You know, the twists, ropes, laces, nibs, jelly beans, whatever the shape from the mass producers. Not licorice.

Seems there is some concern that real licorice elevates blood pressure, so to protect you from the evils of licorice, what you really get now is anise flavoring plus sugar syrup. Somehow that's supposed to be better for us.

Our point is, if you're having a licorice candy to help digestion after your chili dog, you're just doubling down on stupid. "Licorice" isn't helping. You'd get more from a cigarette.

As we just said, there is a compound in real licorice suspected of raising blood pressure. And that leads us to "deglycyrrhizinated" licorice or DGL. These pills, capsules, potions etc. are supposed to be licorice with the bad part removed. Just the good stuff.

Well to start, "deglycyrrhizinated" violates our *Simplify* principle. Nothing benefits from seven syllable communication except maybe obfuscationableness. We made that word up; but someone made up deglycyrrhizinated too. Seven syllables are usually just a way to make the price higher. (Think telecommunications companies. Really? It's just a phone call.)

In general, extracts like DGL violate the *Respect Nature* principle. And the further something gets from its natural state, the more it violates many of our principles: *Respect Nature*, *Simplify*, and *Follow the Money*. Any one of them will help with an evaluation, they all apply here.

If you just chewed the naturally growing licorice plant root like King Tut, it's a pretty fair bet you'd feel better. Maybe even help your reflux too. But be careful, there really is some evidence that too much real licorice increases your blood pressure. That's how we got to the DGL version.

So even after all that principle breaking, we still have to apply our most fundamental *Open Minded* principle here. And there really is some evidence the deglycyrrhizinated licorice product helps with reflux. Mostly subjective, not a lot of hard science behind it, but a lot of people say it helps. It helped us. But no one is exactly sure why.

It is believed that DGL stimulates mucus production in the stomach. And it is believed that it harmonizes many other things happening in there too. Kind of like a catalyst, it makes reactions happen more easily.

Like we said, there is not a lot of hard data, but there is enough anecdotal evidence to take it seriously. More importantly, there is a high probability DGL does no harm. It might work for you, and it can't hurt. DGL helped us, but it was not a "silver bullet" and cannot cure reflux all on its own.

So if you want to pop a pill, try one of the DGL products instead of prescription drugs. They're cheaper, and for some people they work better than the drugs. Even the placebo effect might calm your stomach. Just make sure you get it from a reliable producer. There is not a lot of regulation and there are a lot of rip-offs out there.

Actually, you can't really pop it like a pill. You have to chew it or brew it into a tea. And it tastes like licorice. Real licorice, not sugar syrup, so that might be an eye opener if you're switching from the candies.

Although we don't like seven syllable remedies, we'll give DGL a thumbs up here. It doesn't cost much to try, and the plant its derived from has a long history of providing curative effects. And it can't really hurt anything.

The DontBeStupid.club Summary:

- If you're chewing real licorice root like King Tut, congratulations on *Respecting Nature*.

- DGL is worth a try as long as you trust the supplier.

- And if it's anything else, it's just candy.

- (Find the link to our Amazon store at the very end of the book to find the DGL we like.)

12.
Answer 9: Exercise and Lose Weight?

EVERYONE'S FAVORITE, right? That's why obesity is so rare. We just love to diet and exercise...

We all hate to hear this stuff, so we won't be stupid and just say "you should lose weight and exercise more". We're going to say something similar, but we'll try to make it a more meaningful discussion.

Respect Nature. Your body works better when it moves. (see Answer #2). Your body has to work to maintain whatever load you give it. And losing weight makes that easier.

Statistically, reflux is linked to both a sedentary lifestyle and being overweight. And there is a synergistic effect. The two together actually make it about 3 times more likely you suffer from reflux. That works in reverse too. Eliminate just one and you get more than half the benefits.

So let's work on this overly common advice a little and apply some DontBeStupid.club principles. Maybe everyone can like this answer a little more too. Let's start with strenuous exercise is bad.

Exercise is bad? YAY!!

Wait a minute. Not all exercise, just strenuous. You still have to go for that walk.

But don't expect to be a power-lifter and fight reflux at the same time. Is power lifting contrary to the *Respect Nature* principle? Of course it is. Don't Be Stupid. Humans are not designed to lift multiples of their body weight. You can only train your way into it.

As we keep saying, the body is capable of amazing adaptation. And maybe you can flip a giant tire 10 times. Or even lift the rear end of your car off the ground. And those guys pulling trucks on TV are really fun to watch. But if you're dealing with reflux, you just don't need to do any of that. If you can do a few body weight squats with good form, you will make it through life just fine with a lot less reflux problems.

For all you linebackers who can squat with twice your bodyweight on your shoulders, please don't hate us. We love to watch and are in awe of your physical prowess. Truly. Watching NFL players can be almost scary. But if you're not getting paid enough to put up with reflux, consider the trade-off?

Less strenuous exercise, like Yoga, can be great for you in general, but anti-gravity positions are bad for your reflux. And you don't really want to stand on your head to much anyway, right? We can't quite see how that *Respects Nature* in any case.

Bending over to pick up a heavy weight also defies gravity, and adds straining into the mix at the same time. Bending over to pick up a heavy weight is worse than loading the dishwasher. At least choose weights up on raised racks. And preferably weights you do not have to grunt when you lift. Don't Be Stupid.

The best choice if you're fighting reflux? Explore some

body weight based exercise programs. Pilates, for example, does not require straining if you're doing it right. Leave out the moves that defy gravity, and you can be in great shape without aggravating reflux.

If reflux is your concern, and you are one of the 75% of Americans who exercise less than once a week, consider adding just a minimum workout into your routine: walk a little, do a few body weight squats, and maybe do a few pushups even if only from your knees. Just give your body a little help with pumping every day. A little exercise also reduces your stress level, and that is good for reflux along with a host of other ailments.

On the weight loss part of this remedy, we probably can't say anything new. There are thousands of diet books out there. But let's see if we can apply the *Simplify* principle and cut through the clutter.

First eliminate every diet book you see that has a gimmick. A lot of them are good entertainment, some have food that's fun to eat, some may even help you lose weight. But too many are stupid if taken too seriously. *Follow the Money*. In the end, the gimmicks are there mostly just to extract money from your pocket.

We really hate to endorse websites and are not in the referral business. But *Open Mind*. Sometimes we have to make an exception.

Simplify. Let's just skip to the end. For free, you can simply go to CookingLight.com and get a ton of recipes. Just enter your favorite foods and see what comes up. (We are not affiliated and collect no commission.) This answer is just too easy to ignore.

In general, you are far more likely to lose weight if you still eat food you like. Eating what you like is a force of nature. *Respect Nature*. Plan your diet around what you're going to eat anyway. Build meals and recipes around foods you like. Just don't eat too much (remember Answer #7).

The DontBeStupid.club Summary:

- You can stay in shape with no reflux, just don't over train.

- Staying in shape is cheap medicine; it can be free.

- Losing weight does not have to be torture. Find recipes for foods you like.

- Watch for our DontBeStupid.club books on food, coming soon!

13.
Answer 10: How you Sleep

IF YOU'VE BEEN fighting reflux for a while, then you already know about sleeping on an incline.

A quick explanation for those who are not pros: you spend a long period of time each night in a horizontal position. Gravity neutral. If you can adjust that position to make gravity work for you, it helps.

Now let's get it right because too many people are little stupid here. And this is a good one to get right because it always helps at least a little.

Your body works best when it is approximately straight. It adjusts to being bent and contorted. The body is an amazing machine designed to function under a lot of challenging circumstances. It will tolerate contortions, and let you sleep in all kinds of crazy arrangements. But if you want to heal, help the body out. *Respect Nature*. Keep it straight.

You cannot sleep on extra pillows, or a wedge pillow, or do anything else that bends your body and still gain maximum benefit for reflux.

We tried it. And you or someone you know has tried a wedge pillow or some other way to elevate their head too. Elevating your head actually makes things worse. Your throat can bend when it has to, but it wants to be straight. A lot of people trigger their cough reflex bending their throat. No one helps their reflux by bending their throat.

Movement in that sphincter at the bottom of your throat gets restricted if there are contortions nearby. It can't do its job and acid leaks through. By elevating your head, you just made the sphincter less effective, exactly the opposite of your intention.

Bending your body for sleep violates the *Respect Nature* principle. And you sleep every night. Chances are good you will lose that fight sooner or later. The way to gain maximum benefit is to maintain your body in a single plane, the same as it would be if you were not trying to elevate it for reflux.

A quick *Define the Target*. Plane - the flat surface which wholly contains the line connecting any two points on it. Think of the top of your head as one point and the tip of your toes as the other point on that line. They define the plane your body is in.

You must change the slope of the entire plane in which you sleep. The whole plane, head to toe. The simplest way is to elevate one end of your bed, the end where your head will spend most of the night. You could also shorten the legs at the opposite end. Either way works.

Your body will sleep in the same position it always does. You've just added some slope to the plane. You are adding a little gravity to help keep things going in the right direction, all the way through in the right direction, with no added twists or bends.

You just want a little slope though. You are designed to sleep laying down; you don't get enough rest standing up. 1:30 slope is plenty. That's 3.33%. And if you want it in degrees we're going to talk about inverse-tangents. Nobody else but us really enjoys that? Just raise the head of your bed about 3 inches. Close enough.

If you can, sleep on your left side. This adds a little bonus gravity to your position. The stomach is not symmetrical. It sits a little to your left side. So help things along a little by keeping most of it under your throat. Laying on your right side, you're actually elevating the stomach a little. Try to sleep left.

Do not eat just before sleeping, and try not to take medications or supplements too close to bed time either. *Respect Nature.* Your stomach wants to work on all that stuff with gravity as its ally. Your stomach expects to rest at night just like the rest of you. Don't give it work to do just before you lay down.

Most importantly, sleep well. Sleep is when your body does the most of its healing. And the more your throat heals, the better it will fight off the next blast of reflux that hits it.

The DontBeStupid.club Summary:

- Elevate a little.

- Keep the body straight.

- Sleep on your left side if you can.

- All of this will help with reflux and it doesn't cost anything.

14.
Bonus Answer: Sex

SEX IS FREQUENTLY cited as an acid reflux trigger. And that's stupid.

It violates the *Respect Nature* principle. We are designed to reproduce. If sex caused acid reflux, we'd be extinct. Or at least more scarce. Since the human population is exploding, it's safe to assume sex does not cause reflux.

But there are some correlations that feed this myth.

Eating just before "taking action" can be a problem. Remember the childhood rule about no swimming for an hour after eating? Well... may we suggest a different order of events for date night? Gravity defying positions can cause problems if your stomach is already busy digesting. (Refer to Answer #4).

Stress inducing sex, like maybe you shouldn't be there? That kind of stress will give you acid reflux. Maybe reflux is a force for fidelity.

"Heartburn" is one of the more common side effects of prescription erectile dysfunction drugs. But come on, what man wouldn't trade a little heartburn for a four-hour erection?

Our advice? Do it with someone you love, before dinner, in whatever crazy position works for you. And sometimes before breakfast is good too.

The DontBeStupid.club Summary:

- A summary on sex? Well, we're not stupid.

15.
Closing Remarks

Many more chapters could be written. We discussed the remedies we encountered the most. We've tried all of them, and still use many of them.

Our goal was to help as many people as possible. If we didn't include something specific to you, we hope at least you feel more informed on the topic of reflux in general and maybe better able to think critically about it.

And we hope everyone feels a little more outraged at everyone profiting from the suffering.

If you have an answer we should have included, please let us know. Maybe we'll add it later. Or if we get enough, maybe we'll do a second book. Reflux is a big problem and we know we've only scratched the surface here.

We've tried to keep it light and entertaining while talking about a serious and painful subject. As we said at the start, we feel your pain. But what you just read worked for us and we hope it does for you too.

Our own journey with reflux led through several specialists, including an over-zealous cardiologist who could fix our broken heart. And then we diagnosed the problem and fixed it ourselves. Well, not totally ourselves. We had the help of many well-intentioned people who put many, many ideas out there for consideration.

We just applied ourselves to the task and were not stupid when evaluating all the information. The results are dramatic. Near total relief from a serious problem covering years of suffering. We're ecstatic about it. No more prescriptions and no surgeries.

But we shudder when thinking about all the stupidity we encountered. Unnecessary heart surgeries that may happen because of stupidity? Shudder... Hopefully we prevented one or two here.

There is enough information available to solve most problems, reflux and everything else we ponder over on this earth. The information is out there. It's just that the answers are usually hidden among a lot of stupidity.

The more stupid we are, the more it costs us. Time, anxiety, cash, and frequently pain and suffering too. And Stupidity is BIG business. Everywhere we are stupid, someone else is collecting the cash.

Applying the DontBeStupid.club critical thought process can break this cycle. One topic at a time. We can find answers.

Hopefully we made a contribution here, and we are all a little less stupid about reflux.

16.
Don't Be Stupid Club

At DontBeStupid.club we make the world a little less stupid.

We do not take a position on an issue until we've thought about it critically. We always start with an *Open Mind*. We just apply our principles and think about the question. A little critical thinking is all that's required to quickly reach most answers. Sometimes a little more work is required. But we always get to the answer.

We don't care what people think. But we do care about how they think. Any well-reasoned opinion deserves respect. And opinions without basis are just stupid. Differing answers are fine. All we want is to make the world a little less stupid. If you hate our answer and have a well-reasoned opposition, GREAT!

We're all in this adventure together. We're stupid too. We are all conditioned from birth to think the wrong way. But we are a little less stupid for trying to fix that.

Critical thinking is a skill that can be learned. It's not even a difficult skill. It's harder to be a good welder or good coder or good baseball player. It's impossible for most of us to dunk a basketball. But we all can be good thinkers.

Critical thinking is a way of looking at the world. It's a

framework for thinking about anything. You're going to spend time thinking anyway, why not make the most of it? We think life is easier this way. You never feel lost if you know how to think.

Most disagreements we observe just come from people being stupid. Arguing points without defining their targets... adding complexity to hide their own inadequacies... trying to lie their way to a profit... going against nature... doing the wrong things first... all just stupid.

The world can be a much better place if we are all a little less stupid.

And know this. If you apply our critical thinking principles, then you can never be stupid. The stupidity is all around you, but it can never get YOU! Critical thinking is stronger than stupidity. Answers always equal power.

Our goal is to make a little difference in your life and entertain. Let us know how we did. We'd love to hear from you.

Visit http://DontBeStupid.club if you'd like more.

Our Amazon Store is located at: http://astore.amazon.com/dontbclub-20. It's where you'll find some of the products we like. Nothing in our store is stupid. You don't pay anything extra, but we get a little commission if you buy here. And we appreciate it. It helps us keep making the world a little less stupid.

We thank you for the time you spent with us.

Made in the USA
Lexington, KY
15 April 2016